Unmissable Air Fryer Recipes

Delicious Air Fryer Recipes for Tasty Meals

Kira Hamm

TABLE OF CONTENT

Guacamole 7

Mini Pizza 10

Artichoke with Red Pepper Pizza 12

Artichoke Turkey Pizza 14

Bacon Cheeseburger Pizza 16

Bacon Lettuce Tomato Pizza 18

Breakfast Pizza 20

French Bread Pizza 22

Vegetable Pizza Pan Supreme 24

Garlic Bread Pizza 26

Cheesy Pepperoni Pizza Bites 27

Cheesy BBQ Chicken Pizza 29

Eggplant Pizza 31

Veggie Pizza 33

Grill Pizza Sandwiches 35

Basil Pizza 36

Power XL Air Fryer Pizza Sandwiches 39

Veg Pizza 40

Power XL Air Fryer Grill-baked Grilled Cheese 42

Cheese Chili Toast 43

Cheese Pizza 44

Garlic Bread 45

Pepperoni Pizza	46
Egg Sandwich	47
Grilled Cheese Sandwich	48
Beef and Seeds Burgers	49
Thai Pork Burgers	51
Cheesy Philly Steaks	53
Cheese & Egg Breakfast Sandwich	56
Peanut Butter & Banana Sandwich	57
Super Cheesy Sandwiches	58
Simple Cuban Sandwiches	60
Hot Ham and Cheese Sandwich	62
Philly Cheesesteak Sandwiches	63
Chicken Focaccia Bread Sandwiches	65
Guacamole Turkey Burgers	66
Bread Pudding	68
Cheesy Bread Pudding	70
Chocolate Bread Pudding	72
Fast Pumpkin Pudding	74
Coconut Berry Pudding	76
Pineapple Pudding	77
Cocoa Pudding	78
Cauliflower Pudding	79
Tuna and Lettuce Wraps	80
Crunchy Chicken Egg Rolls	82
Golden Cabbage and Mushroom Spring Rolls	84

Korean Beef and Onion Tacos... 87
Cheesy Sweet Potato and Bean Burritos 89
Golden Chicken and Yogurt Taquitos 92
Cod Tacos with Salsa 94
Golden Spring Rolls 96
Fast Cheesy Bacon and Egg Wraps.. 99
Chicken-Lettuce Wraps..101
Chicken Pita Sandwich...103
Veggie Salsa Wraps...105
Cheesy Shrimp Sandwich 107
Smoky Chicken Sandwich..109

© Copyright 2021 - All rights reserved.

The content contained within this book may not be reproduced, duplicated or transmitted without direct written permission from the author or the publisher.

Under no circumstances will any blame or legal responsibility be held against the publisher, or author, for any damages, reparation, or monetary loss due to the information contained within this book. Either directly or indirectly.

Legal Notice:

This book is copyright protected. This book is only for personal use. You cannot amend, distribute, sell, use, quote or paraphrase any part, or the content within this book, without the consent of the author or publisher.

Disclaimer Notice:

Please note the information contained within this document is for educational and entertainment purposes only. All effort has been executed to present accurate, up to date, and reliable, complete information. No warranties of any kind are declared or implied. Readers acknowledge that the author is not engaging in the rendering of legal, financial, medical or professional advice. The content within this book has been derived from various sources. Please consult a licensed professional before attempting any techniques outlined in this book.

By reading this document, the reader agrees that under no circumstances is the author responsible for any losses, direct or indirect, which are incurred as a result of the use of information contained within this document, including, but not limited to, — errors, omissions, or inaccuracies.

Guacamole

Preparation Time: 15 minutes

Cooking Time: 4 minutes

Servings: 4

Ingredients:

- 2 ripe avocados, halved and pitted
- 2 teaspoons vegetable oil
- 3 tablespoons fresh lime juice
- 1 garlic clove, crushed
- ¼ teaspoon ground chipotle chile
- Salt, as required
- ¼ cup red onion, chopped finely
- ¼ cup fresh cilantro, chopped finely

Directions:

1. Brush the cut sides of each avocado half with oil.
2. Place the water tray in the bottom of Power XL Smokeless Electric Grill.
3. Place about 2 cups of lukewarm water into the water tray.
4. Place the drip pan over water tray and then arrange the heating element.

5. Now, place the grilling pan over heating element.
6. Plugin the Power XL Smokeless Electric Grill and press the 'Power' button to turn it on.
7. Then press 'Fan" button.
8. Set the temperature settings according to manufacturer's Directions:
9. Cover the grill with lid and let it preheat.
10. After preheating, remove the lid and grease the grilling pan.
11. Place the avocado halves over the grilling pan, cut side down.
12. Cook, uncovered for about 2-4 minutes.
13. Transfer the avocados onto cutting board and let them cool slightly.
14. Remove the peel and transfer the flesh into a bowl.
15. Add the lime juice, garlic, chipotle and salt and with a fork, mash until almost smooth.
16. Stir in onion and cilantro and refrigerate, covered for about 1 hour before serving.

Nutrition: Calories 230 Total Fat 21.9 g Saturated Fat 4.6g Cholesterol 0 mg Sodium 46 mg Total Carbs 9.7 g Fiber 6.9 g Sugar 0.8 g Protein 2.1 g

Mini Pizza

Preparation Time 10 minutes

Cooking Time: 20 minutes

Servings: 4

Ingredients:

- 1 tsp of Italian herb seasoning
- 1/4 cup of minced onion
- 6 toasted and split muffins
- 3 tbsp of steak sauce
- 2 cups of mozzarella cheese
- 1/4 cup of sliced green onion
- 1 can of tomato paste
- 3/4 pound of ground beef
- 2 cups of parmesan cheese

Directions:

1. Crumble meat in a bowl, add onion, tomato paste, Italian herb, and steak sauce.
2. Stir well.
3. Spread the mixture on muffins and transfer to the Power XL Air Fryer Grill pan.
4. Set the Power XL Air Fryer Grill to pizza function.

5. Cook for about 20 minutes on both sides at 3500F.
6. Serve immediately with green onions and cheese.
7. Serving Suggestions: Serve with tomato ketchup

Directions: & Cooking Tips: mix the Ingredients: well.

Nutrition: Calories: 273kcal, Fat: 27g, Carb: 23g, Proteins: 21g

Artichoke with Red Pepper Pizza

Preparation Time 10 minutes

Cooking Time: 20 minutes

Serving: 1

Ingredients:

- 1 tsp of dried basil
- 1 can of artichoke hearts
- 1-1/2 cup of mozzarella cheese
- 1 cup of red bell pepper
- 5 cloves of garlic
- Cracked pepper
- 1 tbsp of olive oil
- 1 pizza shell
- 1 tsp of oregano
- 1 jar of sliced mushroom

Directions:

1. Mix artichoke hearts, basil, bell pepper, garlic, and cracked pepper in a bowl.
2. Add oregano, mushroom, and olive oil.
3. Place the mixture on the pizza shell
4. Transfer the pizza shell to Power XL Air Fryer Grill pan.

5. Set the Power XL Air Fryer Grill to pizza function.
6. Cook for about 20 minutes at 3500F.
7. Serve immediately
8. Serving Suggestions: Serve with tomato ketch up
9. Directions: & Cooking Tips: rinse the artichoke well

Nutrition: Calories: 359kcal, Fat: 18g, Carb: 43g, Proteins: 12g

Artichoke Turkey Pizza

Preparation time 10minutes

Cooking Time:10 minutes

Serving: 2

Ingredients:

- 2 cups of chopped cooked turkey
- 1-1/2 cup of mozzarella cheese
- 2 baked pizza crust
- 1 can of black olives
- 1 can of diced tomatoes with garlic, oregano, and basil
- 1/2 cup of shredded parmesan cheese
- 1 can of artichoke hearts

Directions:

1. Place the pizza crusts on a working surface.
2. Place turkey, olive, tomatoes mix, parmesan cheese, olives, and artichokes on them.
3. Transfer the pizza crusts to the Power XL Air Fryer Grill pan.
4. Set the Power XL Air Fryer Grill to pizza function.

5. Cook for 10 minutes at 4500F
6. Serve immediately.
7. Serving Suggestions: Top with mozzarella cheese while serving
8. Directions: & Cooking Tips: drain the heart of the artichoke

Nutrition: Calories: 196kcal, Fat: 7g, Carb: 28g, Proteins: 8g

Bacon Cheeseburger Pizza

Preparation Time 10 minutes

Cooking Time: 10 minutes

Serving: 2

Ingredients:

- 6 bacon strips
- 1/2 pound of ground beef
- 1 tsp of pizza seasoning
- 2 cups of mozzarella cheese
- 2 baked-bread crushes
- 20 slices of dill pickles
- 1 chopped small onion
- 2 cups of shredded cheddar cheese
- 8 ounces of pizza sauce

Directions:

1. Cook onion and beef over medium heat for about 5 minutes.
2. Drain the meat.
3. Add bacon, seasonings, sauce, cheeses, and pickles.
4. Place the bread crusts on a working surface.
5. Place the Ingredients: on them.

6. Transfer it to the Power XL Air Fryer Grill pan
7. Set the Power XL Air Fryer Grill to pizza function.
8. Cook for 10 minutes at 4500F
9. Serving Suggestions: serve with ketchup
10. Directions: & Cooking Tips: rinse the beef and bacon well

Nutrition: Calories: 322kcal, Fat: 12g, Carb: 42g, Proteins: 17g

Bacon Lettuce Tomato Pizza

Preparation and Cooking Time: 10 minutes

Cooking Time: 17 minutes

Serving: 2

Ingredients:

- 6 slices of plum tomatoes
- 1 cup of torn romaine lettuce
- 1/3 cup of mayonnaise
- 8 sliced of bacon
- 2 bread shell
- 1 cup of mozzarella cheese

Directions:

1. Spread the bread shell on a working surface.
2. Put mayonnaise, cheese, bacon, and tomatoes on the bread shells.
3. Transfer to the Power XL Air Fryer Grill pan.
4. Set the Power XL Air Fryer Grill to pizza function.
5. Cook for 17 minutes at 4500F.
6. Serve immediately
7. Serving Suggestions: serve with lettuce

8. Directions: & Cooking Tips: cooked and quartered bacon should be used

Nutrition: Calories: 132kcal, Fat: 8g, Carb: 9g, Proteins: 8g

Breakfast Pizza

Preparation Time: 10 minutes

Cooking Time: 15 minutes

Servings: 5

Ingredients:

- 1 pound of bacon
- 8 ounces of crescent dinner rolls
- 1 cup of cheddar cheese
- 6 eggs

Direction:

1. Place the rolls on the pizza pan.
2. Mix cheese, eggs, and bacon in a bowl.
3. Pour the mixture over the crust.
4. Place the pan in the Power XL Air Fryer Grill.
5. Set the Power XL Air Fryer Grill to pizza function.
6. Cook for 15 minutes at 3700F.
7. Serve immediately
8. Serving Suggestions: serve with ketchup
9. Directions: & Cooking Tips: cooked bacon should be used

Nutrition: Calories: 311kcal, Fat: 11g, Carb: 43g,

Proteins: 15g

French Bread Pizza

Preparation Time: 10 minutes

Cooking Time: 10 minutes

Serving: 4

Ingredients:

- 1 tsp of dried oregano
- 1/2 cup of fresh mushrooms
- 1 loaf of French bread
- 1/4 cup of parmesan cheese
- 1 cup of mozzarella cheese
- 1/2 green pepper
- 3/4 cup of spaghetti sauce

Directions:

1. Put the spaghetti sauce on the French bread.
2. Add green pepper, cheeses, mushroom, and oregano.
3. Place it on the Power XL Air Fryer Grill pan.
4. Set the Power XL Air Fryer Grill to pizza function.
5. Cook for 15 minutes at 3700F.
6. Serving Suggestions: Serve with cheese

7. Directions: & Cooking Tips: shred the mozzarella cheese before using

Nutrition: Calories: 303kcal, Fat: 7g, Carb: 51g, Proteins: 13g

Vegetable Pizza Pan Supreme

Preparation Time: 30 minutes

Cooking Time: 10 Minutes

Servings: 2

Ingredients:

- 1 pizza dough
- 2 tablespoons of olive oil
- 8 creaming mushrooms
- 8 slices of white onion
- 4 tablespoons of pesto
- cup grated mozzarella
- 0.5 green pepper
- 1 cup of spinach
- 12 tomato slices

Directions:

1. Roll the pizza dough halves until each is the size of the airflow shelves.
2. Lightly grease both sides of each dough with olive oil.
3. Place each pizza on a rack. Place the racks on the top and bottom shelves of the Power Air fryer.

4. Press the on/Off button and then the French Fries button (400 ° F) and reduce the cooking Time to 13 minutes.
5. After 5 minutes, turn the dough on the top shelf and rotate the racks.
6. After 4 minutes, turn the dough onto the top shelf.
7. Remove both racks and the top pizzas with toppings.
8. Place the racks on the top and bottom shelves of the electric fryer.
9. Press the power button and then the French fry button (400 ° F) and reduce the cooking Time to 7 minutes.
10. Turn the pizza after 4 minutes.
11. As soon as the pizzas are ready, let them rest for 4 minutes before cutting.

Nutrition: Calories: 183, Carbs: 32.7g, Protein: 9.4g, Fat: 2g.

Garlic Bread Pizza

Preparation Time: 10 minutes

Cooking Time: 10 minutes

Servings: 4

Ingredients:

- 4 pieces baguette, cut in half
- Mint leaves, chopped
- 2-3 tsp. butter
- 2-3 garlic cloves, minced

Directions:

1. Mix butter, mint, and garlic.
2. Spread mixture on every slice.
3. Bake at 200C or 400F in the Power XL Air Fryer Grill for 5-6 minutes

Nutrition: Calories: 160kcal, Carbs: 18g, Protein: 3.6g, Fat: 7.1g.

Cheesy Pepperoni Pizza Bites

Preparation Time: 5 minutes

Cooking Time: 12 minutes

Serves 8

Ingredients:

- 1 cup finely shredded Mozzarella cheese
- ½ cup chopped pepperoni
- ¼ cup Marinara sauce
- 1 (8-ounce) can crescent roll dough
- All-purpose flour, for dusting

Directions:

1. In a small bowl, stir together the cheese, pepperoni, and Marinara sauce.
2. Lay the dough on a lightly floured work surface. Separate it into 4 rectangles. Firmly pinch the perforations together and pat the dough pieces flat.
3. Divide the cheese mixture evenly between the rectangles and spread it out over the dough, leaving a ¼-inch border. Roll a rectangle up tightly, starting with the short

end. Pinch the edge down to seal the roll. Repeat with the remaining rolls.
4. Slice the rolls into 4 or 5 even slices. Place the slices on the sheet pan, leaving a few inches between each slice.
5. Place the pan on the toast position.
6. Select Toast, set temperature to 350°F (180°C) and set Time to 12 minutes.
7. After 6 minutes, rotate the pan and continue cooking.
8. When cooking is complete, the rolls will be golden brown with crisp edges. Remove the pan from the air fryer grill. Serve hot.

Nutrition: Calories: 207cal, Carbs: 17g, Protein: 9g, Fat: 12g.

Cheesy BBQ Chicken Pizza

Preparation Time: 5 minutes

Cooking Time: 8 minutes

Serves 1

Ingredients:

- 1 piece naan bread
- ¼ cup Barbecue sauce
- ¼ cup shredded Monterrey Jack cheese
- ¼ cup shredded Mozzarella cheese
- ½ chicken herby sausage, sliced
- 2 tablespoons red onion, thinly sliced
- Chopped cilantro or parsley, for garnish
- Cooking spray

Directions:

1. Spritz the bottom of naan bread with cooking spray, then transfer to the air fry basket.
2. Brush with the Barbecue sauce. Top with the sausage, cheeses, and finish with the red onion.
3. Place the basket on the air fry position.

4. Select Air Fry, set temperature to 400ºF (205ºC), and set Time to 8 minutes.
5. When cooking is complete, the cheese should be melted. Remove the basket from the air fryer grill. Garnish with the chopped cilantro or parsley before slicing to serve.

Nutrition: Calories: 227cal, Carbs: 18g, Protein: 11g, Fat: 22g.

Eggplant Pizza

Preparation Time: 15 minutes

Cooking Time: 10 minutes

Servings: 2

Ingredients:

- Eggplant (sliced 1/4 -inch)
- Gluten-free pizza dough
- 1 cup of pizza sauce
- Fresh rosemary and basil
- Cheese
- Garlic cloves, chopped
- Red pepper, salt, and pepper
- Olive oil

Directions:

1. Rub eggplant slices with vegetable oil and rosemary, salt and pepper, and bake for 25 mins at 2180C or 4250F in the Power XL Air Fryer Grill.
2. Roll the dough round and spread the remaining Ingredients: on top.

3. Preheat the Power XL Air Fryer Grill at 2300C or 4500F at pizza-setting and bake the pizza for 10 minutes.

Nutrition: Calories: 260kcal, Carbs: 24g, Protein: 9g, Fat 14g.

Veggie Pizza

Preparation Time: 10 minutes

Cooking Time: 10 minutes

Servings: 2

Ingredients:

- 1 cup of tomatoes, sliced
- Capsicum, sliced
- 4 baby corns
- 1-2 tsp. pizza sauce
- 1 cup of mozzarella cheese
- cup of all-purpose flour
- tsp. oregano seasoning
- Salt
- tsp. yeast
- 2-3 tsp. oil
- cup of water

Directions:

1. Make pizza dough with all-purpose flour adding oil, salt, yeast, and water.
2. Spread the remaining Ingredients: on the pizza base made from dough.
3. Preheat the Power XL Air Fryer Grill and bake for 10 minutes.

Nutrition: Calories: 300kcal, Carbs: 37.5g, Protein: 15g, Fat: 10g.

Grill Pizza Sandwiches

Preparation Time: 5 Minutes

Cooking Time: 5 Minutes

Servings: 1

Ingredients:

- 1 French bread sandwich roll, sliced
- 5 tsp. pizza sauce
- 15-20 slices pepperoni
- 1 cup mozzarella cheese, shredded

Directions:

1. Preheat the Power XL Air Fryer Grill to 2500C or 4820F.
2. Spread pizza sauce on the bread.
3. Add toppings, cheese, and pepperoni on each slice of bread.
4. Toast it until the cheese melts.

Nutrition: Calories: 752.1kcal, Carbs: 33.5 g, Protein: 35.2 g, Fat: 15.7g.

Basil Pizza

Preparation Time:10 minutes

Cooking Time: 7 minutes

Servings: 2

Ingredients:

- 1 pizza dough
- 1/2 tablespoon olive oil
- 1 cup pizza sauce
- 11/2 cups part-skim mozzarella cheese, shredded
- 11/2 cups part-skim provolone cheese, shredded
- 10 fresh basil leaves

Directions:

1. Place the water tray in the bottom of Power XL Smokeless Electric Grill.
2. Place about 2 cups of lukewarm water into the water tray.
3. Place the drip pan over water tray and then arrange the heating element.
4. Now, place the grilling pan over heating element.

5. Plugin the Power XL Smokeless Electric Grill and press the 'Power' button to turn it on.
6. Then press 'Fan" button.
7. Set the temperature settings according to manufacturer's Directions:
8. Cover the grill with lid and let it preheat.
9. With your hands, stretch the dough into the size that will fit into the grilling pan.
10. After preheating, remove the lid and grease the grilling pan.
11. Place the dough over the grilling pan.
12. cover with the lid and cook for about 2-3 minutes
13. Remove the lid and with a heat-safe spatula, flip the dough.
14. Cover with the lid and cook for about 2 minutes.
15. Remove the lid and flip the crust.
16. Immediately, spread the pizza sauce over the crust and sprinkle with both kinds of cheese.
17. Cover with the lid and cook for about 1 minute.

18. Remove the lid and cook for about 1 minute or until the cheese is melted.
19. Remove from the grill and immediately top the pizza with basil leaves.
20. Cut into desired sized wedges and serve.

Nutrition: Calories 707 Total Fat 47.5 g Saturated Fat 23.1 g Cholesterol 80 mg Sodium 1000 mg Total Carbs 34.9 g Fiber 3.5 g Sugar 4.6 g Protein 35.8 g

Power XL Air Fryer Pizza Sandwiches

Preparation Time: 5 minutes

Cooking Time: 5minutes

Servings: 1

Ingredients:

- 1 French bread sandwich roll, sliced
- 5 tsp. pizza sauce
- 15-20 slices pepperoni
- 1 cup mozzarella cheese, shredded

Directions:

1. Preheat the Power XL Air Fryer Grill to 2500C or 4820F.
2. Spread pizza sauce on the bread.
3. Add toppings, cheese, and pepperoni on each slice of bread.
4. Toast it until the cheese melts.

Nutrition: Calories: 752.1kcal, Carbs: 33.5 g, Protein: 35.2 g, Fat: 15.7g.

Veg Pizza

Preparation Time: 10 minutes

Cooking Time: 10 minutes

Servings: 2

Ingredients:

- 1 cup tomatoes, sliced
- Capsicum, sliced
- 4 baby corns
- 1-2 tsp. pizza sauce
- 1 cup mozzarella cheese
- cups all-purpose flour
- tsp. oregano seasoning
- Salt
- tsp. yeast
- 2-3 tsp. oil
- cup of water

Directions:

1. Make pizza dough with all-purpose flour adding oil, salt, yeast, and water.
2. Spread the remaining Ingredients: on the pizza base made of dough.
3. Preheat the Power XL Air Fryer Grill and bake for 10 minutes.

Nutrition: Calories: 300kcal, Carbs: 37.5g, Protein: 15g, Fat: 10g.

Power XL Air Fryer Grill-baked Grilled Cheese

Preparation Time: 10 minutes

Cooking Time: 5 minutes

Servings: 1

Ingredients:

- 2 slices bread
- 1-2 tsp. mayonnaise
- 2-3 tsp. cheddar cheese
- Fresh spinach

Directions:

1. Preheat the Power XL Air Fryer Grill to 2000C or 4000F.
2. Spread mayonnaise and cheese on the bread.
3. Bake for 5-7 minutes. Add the spinach.

Nutrition: Calories: 353kcal, Carbs: 42.1g, Protein: 18.9g, Fat: 7.8g.

Cheese Chili Toast

Preparation Time: 5 minutes

Cooking Time: 10 minutes

Servings: 2

Ingredients:

- 2-4 slices bread
- Capsicum, chopped
- Salt & pepper
- 1-2 Chilies
- 20gm cheese, grated
- 10gm cream
- Oil

Directions:

1. Place the bread on the baking pan.
2. Make a mixture of oil, capsicums, peppers, salt, and chilies.
3. Apply the mixture on bread and grated cheese
4. Bake at 180 degrees or 350°F or 177°C for 5-7 minutes in the Power XL Air Fryer Grill. You're all set.

Nutrition: Calories: 135cal, Carbs: 11.6g, Protein: 7.1g, Fat: 6.5g.

Cheese Pizza

Preparation Time: 10 minutes

Cooking Time: 10 minutes

Servings: 4

Ingredients:

- Readymade pizza base
- 2-3 tsp. tomato ketchup
- 100gm cheese, shredded
- Salt & pepper
- 2 ounces mushroom
- Capsicum, onions, tomatoes

Directions:

1. Preheat the Power XL Air Fryer Grill to 2500C or 4820F.
2. Spread ketchup on the pizza base and then toppings and cheese.
3. Bake for 10-12 minutes.

Nutrition: Calories: 306kcal, Carbs: 40g, Protein: 15g, Fat: 11g.

Garlic Bread

Preparation Time: 10 minutes

Cooking Time: 5 minutes

Servings: 4

Ingredients:

- 4 pieces baguette, cut in half
- Mint leaves, chopped
- 2-3 tsp. butter
- 2-3 garlic cloves, minced

Directions:

1. Mix butter, mint, and garlic.
2. Spread mixture on every slice.
3. Bake at 200C or 400F in the Power XL Air Fryer Grill for 5-6 minutes

Nutrition: Calories: 160kcal, Carbs: 18g, Protein: 3.6g, Fat: 7.1g.

Pepperoni Pizza

Preparation Time: 10 minutes

Cooking Time: 10 minutes |

Servings: 8

Ingredients:

- Pepperoni, sliced
- 1 cup pizza sauce
- 1 cup mozzarella cheese
- Readymade pizza dough
- Parmesan cheese, grated

Directions:

1. Arrange toppings on pizza dough.
2. Preheat the Power XL Air Fryer Grill to 1770C or 3500F.
3. Bake for 25 minutes.

Nutrition: Calories: 235kcal, Carbs: 35.6g, Protein: 11g, Fat: 11g.

Egg Sandwich

Preparation Time:10 minutes

Cooking Time: 16 minutes

Servings: 4

Ingredients:

- 4 eggs
- 1 cup light mayonnaise
- 1 tablespoon chopped chives
- Pepper to taste
- 8 slices loaf bread

Direction

1. Add the eggs to the air fryer rack.
2. Select air fry function.
3. Set it to 250 degrees F.
4. Cook for 16 minutes.
5. Place the eggs in a bowl with ice water.
6. Peel and transfer to another bowl.
7. Mash the eggs with a fork.
8. Stir in the mayo, chives and pepper.
9. Spread mixture on bread and top with another bread to make a sandwich.

Nutrition: Calories 121 Fat 20g Protein 9g

Grilled Cheese Sandwich

Preparation Time: 5 minutes

Cooking Time: 8 minutes

Servings: 1

Ingredients:

- 2 slices bread
- 1 tablespoon butter
- 2 slices cheddar cheese

Direction

1. Spread one side of bread slices with butter.
2. Situate the cheese between the two bread slices.
3. Choose grill setting in your air fryer.
4. Cook at 350 degrees F for 5 minutes.
5. Flip and cook for another 3 minutes.

Nutrition: Calories 133 Fat 19g Protein 8g

Beef and Seeds Burgers

Preparation Time: 15 minutes

Cooking Time: 10 minutes

Servings: 4

Ingredients:

- 1 teaspoon cumin seeds
- 1 teaspoon mustard seeds
- 1 teaspoon coriander seeds
- 1 teaspoon dried minced garlic
- 1 teaspoon dried red pepper flakes
- 1 teaspoon kosher salt
- 2 teaspoons ground black pepper
- 1 pound (454 g) 85% lean ground beef
- 2 tablespoons Worcestershire sauce
- 4 hamburger buns
- Mayonnaise, for serving
- Cooking spray

Directions:

1. Spritz the air fry basket with cooking spray.
2. Put the garlic, seeds, salt, red pepper flakes, and ground black pepper in a food

processor. Pulse to ground the mixture coarsely.
3. Put the ground beef in a large bowl. Pour in the seed mixture and drizzle with Worcestershire sauce. Stir to mix well.
4. Divide the mixture into four parts, shape each piece into a ball, and then bash each ball into a patty. Arrange the patties in the basket.
5. Place the basket on the air fry position.
6. Select Air Fry, set temperature to 350ºF (180ºC) and set Time to 10 minutes. Flip the patties with tongs halfway through the cooking Time.
7. When cooked, the patties will be well browned.
8. Assemble the buns with the patties, then drizzle the mayo over the patties to make the burgers. Serve immediately.

Nutrition: Calories 133 Fat 19g Protein 8g

Thai Pork Burgers

Preparation Time: 10 minutes

Cooking Time: 14 minutes

Servings: 6

Ingredients:

- 1 pound (454 g) ground pork
- 1 tablespoon Thai curry paste
- 1 1/2 tablespoons fish sauce
- ¼ cup thinly sliced scallions, white and green parts
- 2 tablespoons minced peeled fresh ginger
- 1 tablespoon light brown sugar
- 1 teaspoon ground black pepper
- 6 slider buns, split open lengthwise, warmed
- Cooking spray

Directions:

1. Spritz the air fry basket with cooking spray.
2. Combine all the ingredients, except for the buns in a large bowl. Stir to mix well.

3. Divide and shape the mixture into six balls, then bash the balls into six 3-inch-diameter patties.
4. Arrange the patties in the basket and spritz with cooking spray.
5. Place the basket on the air fry position.
6. Select Air Fry, set temperature to 375ºF (190ºC) and set Time to 14 minutes. Flip the patties halfway through the cooking Time.
7. When cooked, the patties should be well browned.
8. Assemble the buns with patties to make the sliders and serve immediately.

Nutrition: Calories: 161 protein: 8 g. Fat: 88 g. Carbs: 32 g.

Cheesy Philly Steaks

Preparation Time: 20 minutes

Cooking Time: 20 minutes

Servings: 2

Ingredients:

- 12 ounces (340 g) boneless rib-eye steak, sliced thinly
- 1/2 teaspoon Worcestershire sauce
- 1/2 teaspoon soy sauce
- Kosher salt and ground black pepper, to taste
- 1/2 green bell pepper, stemmed, deseeded, and thinly sliced
- 1/2 small onion, halved and thinly sliced
- 1 tablespoon vegetable oil
- 2 soft hoagie rolls, split three-fourths of the way through
- 1 tablespoon butter, softened
- 2 slices provolone cheese, halved

Directions:

1. Combine the steak, soy sauce, salt, ground black pepper, and Worcestershire sauce in a large bowl. Toss to coat well. Set aside.

2. Combine the bell pepper, onion, vegetable oil, salt, and ground black pepper in a separate bowl. Toss to coat the vegetables well.
3. Pour the steak and vegetables in the air fry basket.
4. Place the basket on the air fry position.
5. Select Air Fry, set temperature to 400ºF (205ºC) and set Time to 15 minutes.
6. When cooked, the steak will be browned and vegetables will be tender. Transfer them on a plate. Set aside.
7. Brush the hoagie rolls with butter and place in the basket.
8. Select Toast and set Time to 3 minutes. Place the basket on the toast position. When done, the rolls should be lightly browned.
9. Transfer the rolls to a clean work surface and divide the steak and vegetable mix between the rolls. Spread with cheese. Place the stuffed rolls back in the basket.
10. Place the basket on the air fry position.

11. Select Air Fry and set Time to 2 minutes. When done, the cheese should be melted.
12. Serve immediately.

Nutrition : Calories: 1564 kcal Carbs: 9g Fat: 3.5g Protein: 8.6g

Cheese & Egg Breakfast Sandwich

Preparation Time: 3 Minutes

Cooking Time: 6 Minutes

Servings: 1

Ingredients:

- One egg
- Two slices of cheddar or Swiss cheese
- A bit of butter
- One roll either English muffin or Kaiser bun halved

Directions:

1. Butter the sliced rolls on both sides.
2. Whisk the eggs in an oven-safe dish.
3. Place the cheese, egg dish, and rolls into the air fryer. Make sure the buttered sides of the roll are facing upwards.
4. Adjust the air fryer to 390 F. Cook for 6 minutes.
5. Place the egg and cheese between the pieces of roll. Serve warm.

Nutrition: Calories: 212 kcal Total Fat: 11.2g Carbs: 9.3g Protein: 12.4g

Peanut Butter & Banana Sandwich

Preparation Time: 4 Minutes

Cooking Time: 6 Minutes

Servings: 1

Ingredients:

- 2 slices whole-wheat bread
- 1 tsp. sugar-free maple syrup
- One sliced banana
- 2 tbsps. peanut butter

Directions:

1. Evenly coat each side of the sliced bread with peanut butter.
2. Add the sliced banana and drizzle with some sugar-free maple syrup.
3. Adjust the air fryer to 330 F, then cook for 6 minutes. Serve warm.

Nutrition: Calories: 211 kcal Total Fat: 8.2g Carbs: 6.3g Protein: 11.2g

Super Cheesy Sandwiches

Preparation Time: 10 minutes

Cooking Time: 6 minutes

Serves 4 to 8

Ingredients:

- 8 ounces Brie
- 8 slices oat nut bread
- 1 large ripe pear, cored and cut into ½-inch-thick slices
- 2 tablespoons butter, melted

Directions:

1. Make the sandwiches: Spread each of 4 slices of bread with ¼ of the Brie. Top the Brie with the pear slices and remaining 4 bread slices.
2. Brush the melted butter lightly on both sides of each sandwich.
3. Arrange the sandwiches in the air fry basket.
4. Place the basket on the bake position.
5. Select Bake, set temperature to 360°F (182°C), and set Time to 6 minutes.

6. When cooking is complete, the cheese should be melted. Remove the basket from the air fryer grill and serve warm.

Nutrition: Calories: 154 kcal Carbs: 9g Fat: 2.5g Protein: 8.6g

Simple Cuban Sandwiches

Preparation Time: 20 minutes

Cooking Time: 8 minutes

Makes 4 sandwiches

Ingredients:

- slices ciabatta bread, about ¼-inch thick
- Cooking spray
- 1 tablespoon brown mustard
- Toppings:
- 6 to 8 ounces thinly sliced leftover roast pork
- 4 ounces thinly sliced deli turkey
- 1/3 cup bread and butter pickle slices
- 2 to 3 ounces Pepper Jack cheese slices

Directions:

1. On a clean work surface, spray one side of each slice of bread with cooking spray. Spread the other side of each slice of bread evenly with brown mustard.
2. Top 4 of the bread slices with the turkey, roast pork, pickle slices, cheese, and finish

with remaining bread slices. Transfer to the air fry basket.

3. Place the basket on the air fry position.
4. Select Air Fry, set temperature to 390ºF (199ºC), and set Time to 8 minutes.
5. When cooking is complete, remove the basket from the air fryer grill. Cool for 5 minutes and serve warm.

Nutrition: Calories: 164 kcal Carbs: 10g Fat: 4.5g Protein: 8.7g

Hot Ham and Cheese Sandwich

Preparation Time: 5 minutes

Cooking Time: 10 minutes

Servings: 2

Ingredients:

- 2-4 sandwich bread
- Olive oil
- 1/4 tsp. oregano & basil
- 4 ounces ham, sliced
- 4 ounces cheese, sliced

Directions:

1. Preheat the Power XL Air Fryer Grill to 2000C or 4000F.
2. Apply vegetable oil and sprinkle oregano on each side of bread slices.
3. Put the ham, spread cheese over one bread slice, and place the opposite on the sheet.
4. Bake for 10 minutes.

Nutrition: Calories: 245kcal, Carbs: 28g, Protein: 16.18g, Fat: 18.53g.

Philly Cheesesteak Sandwiches

Preparation Time: 15 minutes

Cooking Time: 15 minutes

Servings: 6

Ingredients:

- 1-2 pounds steak
- 1 tsp. Worcestershire sauce
- Salt & pepper
- 2 tsp. butter
- 1 green bell pepper
- Cheese slices
- Bread rolls

Directions:

1. Marinate the steak with sauce, pepper, and salt. Cook the steak in a pan with butter until brown.
2. Cook veggies for 2-3 mins
3. Slice steak and place it on bread rolls with veggies, sliced cheese, and bell peppers.
4. Bake for a quarter-hour in the Power XL Air Fryer Grill.

Nutrition: Calories: 476kcal, Carbs: 15g, Protein:

37g, Fat: 35g.

Chicken Focaccia Bread Sandwiches

Preparation Time 15 minutes

Cooking Time: 25 minutes

Servings: 6

Ingredients:

- Flatbread or Focaccia, halved
- 2 cups of chicken, sliced
- Fresh basil leaves
- 1 cup of sweet pepper, roasted

Directions:

1. Roast the chicken at 1770C or 3500F in the Power XL Air Fryer Grill for 25 to half-hour.
2. Spread mayonnaise on the bread and put the remaining Ingredients: on top.

Nutrition: Calories: 263cal, Carbs: 26.9g, Protein: 19g, Fat: 10g.

Guacamole Turkey Burgers

Preparation Time: 10 Minutes

Cooking Time: 30 minutes

Servings: 3

Ingredients:

- 12 oz. turkey, ground
- 1-1/2 avocados
- 2 teaspoons of juice from a lime
- ½ teaspoon cumin
- 1 red chili, chopped
- ½ teaspoon garlic powder
- ½ teaspoon onion powder
- 3 teaspoons of olive oil
- ½ teaspoon salt

Directions:

1. Mix the turkey with the cumin, chili, salt, garlic powder, and onion powder in a medium-sized bowl.
2. Create 3 patties
3. Pour 3 teaspoons olive oil in a skillet and heat over medium heat.
4. Now cook your patties. Make sure that both sides are brown.

5. Make the guacamole in the meantime.
6. Mash together the garlic powder, juice from lime and avocados in a bowl.
7. Add salt for seasoning.
8. Serve the burgers with guacamole on the patties.

Nutrition : Calories 316, Carbohydrates 9g, Fiber 8g, Sugar 0g, Cholesterol 80mg, Total Fat 21g, Protein 24g

Bread Pudding

Preparation Time 10 minutes

Cooking Time:1 hour

Serving: 8

Ingredients:

- 3 eggs
- 2 tbsp of vanilla
- 3 cups of whole milk
- 3 egg yolks
- 2 tsp of cinnamon
- 8 tbsp of butter
- 1 cups of cubed French bread
- 2 cups of granulated sugar
- 1/4 pyrex bowl

Directions:

1. Mix milk and butter in a bowl and heat in the microwave.
2. Break the egg in another bowl and whisk.
3. Add cinnamon, sugar, eggs, and vanilla.
4. Add the milk mix.
5. Add dried bread, mix until the bread is soaked.
6. Put the mixture in a pyrex bowl

7. Place the pyrex bowl on the Power XL Air Fryer Grill pan.
8. Set the Power XL Air Fryer Grill to bagel/toast.
9. Cook 60 minutes at 2700F.
10. Allow cooling before serving
11. Serving Suggestions: Serve with Cointreau sauce
12. Directions: & Cooking Tips: dried bread should be used

Nutrition: Calories: 379kcal, Fat: 8g, Carb: 70g, Proteins: 9g

Cheesy Bread Pudding

Preparation Time 10 minutes

Cooking Time: 8 minutes

Serving: 4

Ingredients:

- 4 cloves of garlic
- 1 cup of mozzarella cheese
- 8 slices of bread
- 6 tsp of sun-dried tomatoes
- 5 tbsp of melted butter

Directions:

1. Place the bread slices on a flat surface.
2. Put butter on it, garlic, and tomato paste.
3. Add cheese
4. Place the bread on the Power XL Air Fryer Grill pan.
5. Set the Power XL Air Fryer Grill to toast/bagel function.
6. Cook for 8 minutes a 3500F.
7. Serving Suggestions: Can be served with orange juice
8. Directions: & Cooking Tips: Directions: are with tomato paste.

Nutrition: Calories: 226kcal, Fat: 8g, Carb: 32g, Proteins: 8g

Chocolate Bread Pudding

Preparation Time: 10 minutes

Cooking Time: 10 minutes

Serves 8

Ingredients:

- 1 egg
- 1 egg yolk
- ¾ cup chocolate milk
- 3 tablespoons brown sugar
- 3 tablespoons peanut butter
- 2 tablespoons cocoa powder
- 1 teaspoon vanilla
- 5 slices firm white bread, cubed
- Nonstick cooking spray

Directions:

1. Spritz a baking pan with nonstick cooking spray.
2. Whisk together the egg yolk, egg, peanut butter, chocolate milk, cocoa powder, brown sugar, and vanilla until well combined.
3. Fold in the bread cubes and stir to mix well. Allow the bread soak for 10 minutes.

4. When ready, transfer the egg mixture to the baking pan.
5. Place the pan on the bake position.
6. Select Bake, set temperature to 330ºF (166ºC), and set Time to 10 minutes.
7. When done, the pudding should be just firm to the touch.
8. Serve at room temperature.

Nutrition: Calories: 164 Protein: 2 g. Fat: 22 g. Carbs: 4 g.

Fast Pumpkin Pudding

Preparation Time: 10 minutes

Cooking Time: 15 minutes

Serves 4

Ingredients:

- 1 cup canned no-salt-added pumpkin purée (not pumpkin pie filling)
- ¼ cup packed brown sugar
- 3 tablespoons all-purpose flour
- 1 egg, whisked
- 2 tablespoons milk
- 1 tablespoon unsalted butter, melted
- 1 teaspoon pure vanilla extract
- 4 low-fat vanilla wafers, crumbled
- Cooking spray

Directions:

1. Coat a baking pan with cooking spray. Set aside.
2. Mix the pumpkin purée, flour, brown sugar, whisked egg, melted butter, milk, and vanilla in a medium bowl and whisk to combine. Transfer the mixture to the baking pan.

3. Place the pan on the bake position.
4. Select Bake, set temperature to 350ºF (180ºC), and set Time to 15 minutes.
5. When cooking is complete, the pudding should be set.
6. Remove the pudding from the air fryer grill to a wire rack to cool.
7. Divide the pudding into four bowls and serve with the vanilla wafers sprinkled on top.

Nutrition: Calories: 184 Protein: 2 g. Fat: 12 g. Carbs: 3 g.

Coconut Berry Pudding

Preparation Time: 10 minutes

Cooking Time: 15 minutes

Servings: 6

Ingredients:

- 2 cups coconut cream
- 1 lime zest, grated
- 3 tbsp erythritol
- ¼ cup blueberries
- 1/3 cup blackberries

Directions:

1. Add all Ingredients into the blender and blend until well combined.
2. Spray 6 ramekins with cooking spray.
3. Pour blended mixture into the ramekins and place in the air fryer.
4. Cook at 340 F for 15 minutes.
5. Serve and enjoy.

Nutrition: Calories: 164 Protein: 2 g. Fat: 22 g. Carbs: 4 g.

Pineapple Pudding

Preparation Time: 10 Minutes

Cooking Time: 5 Minutes

Servings: 8

Ingredients:

- 1 tablespoon avocado oil
- 1 cup rice
- 14ounces milk
- Sugar to the taste
- 8ounces canned pineapple, chopped

Directions:

1. In your air fryer, mix oil, milk and rice, stir, cover and cook on High for 3 minutes.
2. Add sugar and pineapple, stir, cover and cook on High for 2 minutes more.
3. Divide into dessert bowls and serve.

Nutrition: Calories: 154 Protein: 8 g. Fat: 4 g. Carbs: 14 g.

Cocoa Pudding

Preparation Time: 10 Minutes

Cooking Time: 20 Minutes

Servings: 2

Ingredients:

- 2 tablespoons water
- 1/2 tablespoon agar
- 4 tablespoons stevia
- 4 tablespoons cocoa powder
- 2 cups coconut milk, hot

Directions:

1. In a bowl, mix milk with stevia and cocoa powder and stir well.
2. In a bowl, mix agar with water, stir well, add to the cocoa mix, stir and transfer to a pudding pan that fits your air fryer.
3. Introduce in the fryer and cook at 356 degrees F for 20 minutes.
4. Serve the pudding cold.
5. Enjoy!

Nutrition: Calories: 170 Protein: 3 g. Fat: 2 g. Carbs: 4 g.

Cauliflower Pudding

Preparation Time: 10 Minutes

Cooking Time: 30 Minutes

Servings: 4

Ingredients:

- 2 1/2 cups water
- 1 cup coconut sugar
- 2 cups cauliflower rice
- 2 cinnamon sticks
- 1/2 cup coconut, shredded

Directions:

1. In a pot that fits your air fryer, mix water with coconut sugar, cauliflower rice, cinnamon and coconut, stir, introduce in the fryer and cook at 365 degrees F for 30 minutes
2. Divide pudding into cups and serve cold. Enjoy!

Nutrition: Calories: 203 Protein: 4 g. Fat: 4 g. Carbs: 9 g.

Tuna and Lettuce Wraps

Preparation Time: 10 minutes

Cooking Time: 4 to 7 minutes

Servings: 4

Ingredients:

- 1 pound (454 g) fresh tuna steak, cut into 1-inch cubes
- 1 tablespoon grated fresh ginger
- 2garlic cloves, minced
- ½ teaspoon toasted sesame oil
- 2low-sodium whole-wheat tortillas
- ¼ cup low-fat mayonnaise
- 1cups shredded romaine lettuce
- 1 red bell pepper, thinly sliced

Directions:

1. In a medium bowl, mix the tuna, ginger, garlic, and sesame oil. Let it stand for 10 minutes.
2. Transfer the tuna to the air fryer basket.
3. Select the Air Fry function and cook at 390 degrees Fahrenheit (199 degrees Celsius) for 4 to 7 minutes, or until lightly browned.

4. Make the wraps with the tuna, tortillas, mayonnaise, lettuce, and bell pepper.
5. Serve immediately.

Nutrition : Calories 485 Carbohydrates 6.3g Protein 47.6g Fat 29.9g

Crunchy Chicken Egg Rolls

Preparation Time: 10 minutes

Cooking Time: 24 minutes

Servings: 4

Ingredients:

- 1 pound (454 g) ground chicken
- 2 teaspoons olive oil
- 2 garlic cloves, minced
- 1 teaspoon grated fresh ginger
- 2 cups white cabbage, shredded
- 1 onion, chopped
- ¼ cup soy sauce
- 8 egg roll wrappers
- 1 egg, beaten
- Cooking spray

Directions:

1. Spritz the air fry basket with cooking spray.
2. Heat olive oil in a saucepan over medium heat. Sauté the garlic and ginger in the olive oil for 1 minute, or until fragrant. Add the ground chicken to the saucepan. Sauté

for 5 minutes, or until the chicken is cooked through. Add the cabbage, onion and soy sauce and sauté for 5 to 6 minutes, or until the vegetables become soft. Remove the saucepan from the heat.
3. Unfold the egg roll wrappers on a clean work surface. Divide the chicken mixture among the wrappers and brush the edges of the wrappers with the beaten egg. Tightly roll up the egg rolls, enclosing the filling. Arrange the rolls in the basket.
4. Place the basket on the air fry position.
5. Select Air Fry, set temperature to 370ºF (188ºC) and set Time to 12 minutes. Flip the rolls halfway through the cooking Time.
6. When cooked, the rolls will be crispy and golden brown.
7. Transfer to a platter and let cool for 5 minutes before serving.

Nutrition: Calories: 181 protein: 3 g. Fat: 98 g. Carbs: 42 g.

Golden Cabbage and Mushroom Spring Rolls

Preparation Time: 20 minutes

Cooking Time: 14 minutes

Servings: 14

Ingredients:

- 2 tablespoons vegetable oil - 4 cups sliced Napa cabbage
- 5 ounces (142 g) shiitake mushrooms, diced
- 3 carrots, cut into thin matchsticks
- 1 tablespoon minced fresh ginger
- 1 tablespoon minced garlic
- 1 bunch scallions, white and light green parts only, sliced
- 2 tablespoons soy sauce
- 1 (4-ounce / 113-g) package cellophane noodles
- ¼ teaspoon cornstarch
- 1 (12-ounce / 340-g) package frozen spring roll wrappers, thawed
- Cooking spray

Directions:

1. Heat the olive oil in a nonstick skillet over medium-high heat until shimmering.
2. Add the cabbage, carrots, and mushrooms and sauté for 3 minutes or until tender.
3. Add the garlic, scallions, and ginger and sauté for 1 minutes or until fragrant.
4. Mix in the soy sauce and turn off the heat. Discard any liquid remains in the skillet and allow to cool for a few minutes.
5. Bring a pot of water to a boil, then turn off the heat and pour in the noodles. Let sit for 10 minutes or until the noodles are al dente. Transfer 1 cup of the noodles in the skillet and toss with the cooked vegetables. Reserve the remaining noodles for other use.
6. Dissolve the cornstarch in a small water dish, then place the wrappers on a clean work surface. Dab the edges of the wrappers with cornstarch.
7. Scoop up 3 tablespoons of filling in the center of each wrapper, then fold the corner in front of you over the filling. Tuck the wrapper under the filling, then fold the

corners on both sides into the center. Keep rolling to seal the wrapper. Repeat with remaining wrappers. Spritz the air fry basket with cooking spray. Arrange the wrappers in the basket and spritz with cooking spray.

8. Place the basket on the air fry position.
9. Select Air Fry, set temperature to 400ºF (205ºC) and set Time to 10 minutes. Flip the wrappers halfway through the cooking Time.
10. When cooking is complete, the wrappers will be golden brown.
11. Serve immediately.

Nutrition : Calories: 161 protein: 8 g. Fat: 88 g. Carbs: 32 g.

Korean Beef and Onion Tacos

Preparation Time: 1 hour 15 minutes

Cooking Time: 12 minutes

Servings: 6

Ingredients:

- 2 tablespoons gochujang
- 1 tablespoon soy sauce
- 2 tablespoons sesame seeds
- 2 teaspoons minced fresh ginger
- 2 cloves garlic, minced
- 2 tablespoons toasted sesame oil
- 2 teaspoons sugar
- 1/2 teaspoon kosher salt
- 11/2 pounds (680 g) thinly sliced beef chuck
- 1 medium red onion, sliced
- 6 corn tortillas, warmed
- ¼ cup chopped fresh cilantro
- 1/2 cup kimchi
- 1/2 cup chopped green onions

Directions:

1. Combine the ginger, garlic, gochujang, sesame seeds, soy sauce, sesame oil, salt, and sugar in a large bowl. Stir to mix well.
2. Dunk the beef chunk in the large bowl. Press to submerge, then wrap the bowl in plastic and refrigerate to marinate for at least 1 hour.
3. Remove the beef chunk from the marinade and transfer to the air fry basket. Add the onion to the basket.
4. Place the basket on the air fry position.
5. Select Air Fry, set temperature to 400ºF (205ºC) and set Time to 12 minutes. Stir the mixture halfway through the cooking Time.
6. When cooked, the beef will be well browned.
7. Unfold the tortillas on a clean work surface, divide the fried beef and onion on the tortillas. Spread the green onions, kimchi, and cilantro on top.
8. Serve immediately.

Nutrition: Calories: 181 protein: 3 g. Fat: 98 g. Carbs: 42 g.

Cheesy Sweet Potato and Bean Burritos

Preparation Time: 15 minutes

Cooking Time: 30 minutes

Servings: 6

Ingredients:

- 2 sweet potatoes, peeled and cut into a small dice
- 1 tablespoon vegetable oil
- Kosher salt and ground black pepper, to taste
- 6 large flour tortillas
- 1 (16-ounce / 454-g) can refried black beans, divided
- 1 1/2 cups baby spinach, divided
- 6 eggs, scrambled
- ¾ cup grated Cheddar cheese, divided
- ¼ cup salsa
- ¼ cup sour cream
- Cooking spray

Directions :

1. Put the sweet potatoes in a large bowl, then drizzle with vegetable oil and sprinkle with salt and black pepper. Toss to coat well.
2. Place the potatoes in the air fry basket.
3. Place the basket on the air fry position.
4. Select Air Fry, set temperature to 400°F (205°C) and set Time to 10 minutes. Flip the potatoes halfway through the cooking Time.
5. When done, the potatoes should be lightly browned. Remove the potatoes from the air fryer grill.
6. Unfold the tortillas on a clean work surface. Divide the air fried sweet potatoes, black beans, spinach, scrambled eggs, and cheese on top of the tortillas.
7. Fold the long side of the tortillas over the filling, then fold in the shorter side to wrap the filling to make the burritos.
8. Wrap the burritos in the aluminum foil and put in the basket.
9. Place the basket on the air fry position.
10. Select Air Fry, set temperature to 350°F (180°C) and set Time to 20 minutes. Flip

the burritos halfway through the cooking Time.

11. Remove the burritos from the air fryer grill and spread with sour cream and salsa. Serve immediately.

Nutrition : Calories 133 Fat 19g Protein 8g

Golden Chicken and Yogurt Taquitos

Preparation Time: 15 minutes

Cooking Time: 12 minutes

Servings: 4

Ingredients:

- 1 cup cooked chicken, shredded
- ¼ cup Greek yogurt
- ¼ cup salsa
- 1 cup shredded Mozzarella cheese
- Salt and ground black pepper, to taste
- 4 flour tortillas
- Cooking spray

Directions:

1. Spritz the air fry basket with cooking spray.
2. Combine all the ingredients, except for the tortillas, in a large bowl. Stir to mix well.
3. Make the taquitos: Unfold the tortillas on a clean work surface, then scoop up 2 tablespoons of the chicken mixture in the middle of each tortilla. Roll the tortillas up to wrap the filling.

4. Arrange the taquitos in the basket and spritz with cooking spray.
5. Place the basket on the air fry position.
6. Select Air Fry, set temperature to 380°F (193°C) and set Time to 12 minutes. Flip the taquitos halfway through the cooking Time.
7. When cooked, the taquitos should be golden brown and the cheese should be melted.
8. Serve immediately.

Nutrition : Calories 153 Fat 15g Protein 9g

Cod Tacos with Salsa

Preparation Time: 5 minutes

Cooking Time: 15 minutes

Servings: 4

Ingredients:

- 2 eggs
- 1¼ cups Mexican beer
- 11/2 cups coconut flour
- 11/2 cups almond flour
- 1/2 tablespoon chili powder
- 1 tablespoon cumin
- Salt, to taste
- 1 pound (454 g) cod fillet, slice into large pieces
- 4 toasted corn tortillas
- 4 large lettuce leaves, chopped
- ¼ cup salsa
- Cooking spray

Directions:

1. Spritz the air fry basket with cooking spray.
2. Break the eggs in a bowl, then pour in the beer. Whisk to combine well.

3. Combine the almond flour, coconut flour, cumin, chili powder, and salt in a separate bowl. Stir to mix well.
4. Dunk the cod pieces in the egg mixture, then shake the excess off and dredge into the flour mixture to coat well. Arrange the cod in the basket.
5. Place the basket on the air fry position.
6. Select Air Fry, set temperature to 375ºF (190ºC) and set Time to 15 minutes. Flip the cod halfway through the cooking Time.
7. When cooking is complete, the cod should be golden brown.
8. Unwrap the toasted tortillas on a large plate, then divide the cod and lettuce leaves on top. Baste with salsa and wrap to serve.

Nutrition: Calories 133 Fat 19g Protein 8g

Golden Spring Rolls

Preparation Time: 10 minutes

Cooking Time: 18 minutes

Servings: 4

Ingredients:

- 4 spring roll wrappers
- 1/2 cup cooked vermicelli noodles
- 1 teaspoon sesame oil
- 1 tablespoon freshly minced ginger
- 1 tablespoon soy sauce
- 1 clove garlic, minced
- 1/2 red bell pepper, deseeded and chopped
- 1/2 cup chopped carrot
- 1/2 cup chopped mushrooms
- ¼ cup chopped scallions
- Cooking spray

Directions:

1. Spritz the air fry basket with cooking spray and set aside.
2. Heat the sesame oil in a saucepan on medium heat. Sauté the garlic and ginger in the sesame oil for 1 minute, or until

fragrant. Add soy sauce, carrot, red bell pepper, mushrooms and scallions. Sauté for 5 minutes or until the vegetables become tender. Mix in vermicelli noodles. Turn off the heat and remove them from the saucepan. Allow to cool for 10 minutes.

3. Lay out one spring roll wrapper with a corner pointed toward you. Scoop the noodle mixture on spring roll wrapper and fold corner up over the mixture. Fold left and right corners toward the center and continue to roll to make firmly sealed rolls.
4. Arrange the spring rolls in the basket and spritz with cooking spray.
5. Place the basket on the air fry position.
6. Select Air Fry, set temperature to 340ºF (171ºC) and set Time to 12 minutes. Flip the spring rolls halfway through the cooking Time.
7. When done, the spring rolls will be golden brown and crispy.
8. Serve warm.

Nutrition: Calories 137 Fat 15g Protein 10g

Fast Cheesy Bacon and Egg Wraps

Preparation Time: 15 minutes

Cooking Time: 10 minutes

Servings: 3

Ingredients:

- 3 corn tortillas
- 3 slices bacon, cut into strips
- 2 scrambled eggs
- 3 tablespoons salsa
- 1 cup grated Pepper Jack cheese
- 3 tablespoons cream cheese, divided
- Cooking spray

Directions:

1. Spritz the air fry basket with cooking spray.
2. Unfold the tortillas on a clean work surface, divide the bacon and eggs in the middle of the tortillas, and then spread with scatter and salsa with cheeses. Fold the tortillas over.
3. Arrange the tortillas in the basket.
4. Place the basket on the air fry position.

5. Select Air Fry, set temperature to 390ºF (199ºC) and set Time to 10 minutes. Flip the tortillas halfway through the cooking Time.
6. When cooking is complete, the cheeses will be melted and the tortillas will be lightly browned.
7. Serve immediately.

Nutrition: Calories 133 Fat 19g Protein 8g

Chicken-Lettuce Wraps

Preparation Time: 15 minutes

Cooking Time: 12 to 16 minutes

Servings: 2 to 4

Ingredients:

- 1 pound (454 g) boneless, skinless chicken thighs, trimmed
- 1 teaspoon vegetable oil
- tablespoons lime juice
- 1 shallot, minced
- 1 tablespoon fish sauce, plus extra for serving
- 1teaspoons packed brown sugar
- 1 garlic clove, minced
- 1/8teaspoon red pepper flakes
- 1 mango, peeled, pitted, and cut into 1/4inch pieces
- 1/3 cup chopped fresh mint
- 1/3cup chopped fresh cilantro
- 1/3 cup chopped fresh Thai basil
- 1 head Bibb lettuce, leaves separated (8 ounces / 227 g)
- 1/4cup chopped dry-roasted peanuts

- Thai chiles, stemmed and sliced thin

Directions:

1. Pat the chicken dry with paper towels and rub with oil. Place the chicken in air fryer basket. Select the Air Fry function and cook at 400 degrees Fahrenheit (204 degrees Celsius) for 12 to 16 minutes, or until the chicken registers 175 degrees Fahrenheit (79 degrees Celsius), flipping and rotating chicken halfway through cooking.
2. Meanwhile, whisk lime juice, shallot, fish sauce, sugar, garlic, and pepper flakes together in large bowl; set aside.
3. Transfer chicken to cutting board, let cool slightly, then shred into bite-size pieces using 2 forks. Add the shredded chicken, mango, mint, cilantro, and basil to bowl with dressing and toss to coat.
4. Serve the chicken in the lettuce leaves, passing peanuts, Thai chiles, and extra fish sauce separately.

Nutrition : Calories 311 Fat 11g Carbohydrate 22g Protein 31g

Chicken Pita Sandwich

Preparation Time: 10 minutes

Cooking Time: 9 to 11 minutes

Servings: 4

Ingredients:

- 2 boneless, skinless chicken breasts, cut into 1-inch cubes
- 1 small red onion, sliced
- 1 red bell pepper, sliced
- 1/3 cup Italian salad dressing, divided
- 1/2 teaspoon dried thyme
- 4 pita pockets, split
- 2 cups torn butter lettuce
- 1 cup chopped cherry tomatoes

Directions:

1. Select the Bake function and preheat Maxx to 380 degrees Fahrenheit (193 degrees Celsius).
2. Place the chicken, onion, and bell pepper in the air fryer basket. Drizzle with 1 tablespoon of the Italian salad dressing, add the thyme, and toss.

3. Bake for 9 to 11 minutes, or until the chicken is 165 degrees Fahrenheit (74 degrees Celsius) on a food thermometer, stirring once during cooking Time.
4. Transfer the chicken and vegetables to a bowl and toss with the remaining salad dressing.
5. Assemble sandwiches with the pita pockets, butter lettuce, and cherry tomatoes. Serve immediately.

Nutrition : Calories 311 Fat 11g Carbohydrate 22g Protein 31g

Veggie Salsa Wraps

Preparation Time: 5 minutes

Cooking Time: 7 minutes

Servings: 4

Ingredients:

- 1 cup red onion, sliced
- 1 zucchini, chopped
- 1 poblano pepper, deseeded and finely chopped
- 1 head lettuce
- ½ cup salsa
- 8ounces (227 g) Mozzarella cheese

Directions:

1. Place the red onion, zucchini, and poblano pepper in the air fryer basket. Select the Air Fry function and cook at 390 degrees Fahrenheit (199 degrees Celsius) for 7 minutes, or until they are tender and fragrant.
2. Divide the veggie mixture among the lettuce leaves and spoon the salsa over the top. Finish off with Mozzarella cheese. Wrap the lettuce leaves around the filling.

3. Serve immediately.

Nutrition : Calories 140 Fat 4g Fiber 3g Carbohydrates 5g Protein 7g

Cheesy Shrimp Sandwich

Preparation Time: 10 minutes

Cooking Time: 5 to 7 minutes

Servings: 4

Ingredients:

- 1¼ cups shredded Colby, Cheddar, or Havarti cheese
- 1 (6-ounce / 170-g) can tiny shrimp, drained
- 3 tablespoons mayonnaise
- 2 tablespoons minced green onion
- 4 slices whole grain or whole-wheat bread
- 2 tablespoons softened butter

Directions:

1. In a medium bowl, combine the cheese, shrimp, mayonnaise, and green onion, and mix well.
2. Spread this mixture on two of the slices of bread. Top with the other slices of bread to make two sandwiches. Spread the sandwiches lightly with butter.
3. Select the Air Fry function and cook at 400 degrees Fahrenheit (204 degrees Celsius)

for 5 to 7 minutes, or until the bread is browned and crisp and the cheese is melted.

4. Cut in half and serve warm.

Nutrition: Calories 602 Fat 23.9g Carbohydrates 46.5g Sugar 2.9g Protein 11.3g Sodium 886mg

Smoky Chicken Sandwich

Preparation Time: 10 minutes

Cooking Time: 11 minutes

Servings: 2

Ingredients:

- 2 boneless, skinless chicken breasts (8 ounces / 227 g each), sliced horizontally in half and separated into 4 thinner cutlets
- Kosher salt and freshly ground black pepper, to taste
- ½ cup all-purpose flour
- 3 large eggs, lightly beaten
- ½ cup dried bread crumbs
- 1 tablespoon smoked paprika
- Cooking spray
- ½ cup marinara sauce
- 6 ounces (170 g) smoked Mozzarella cheese, grated
- 2 store-bought soft, sesame-seed hamburger or Italian buns, split

Directions:

1. Season the chicken cutlets all over with salt and pepper. Set up three shallow bowls:

Place the flour in the first bowl, the eggs in the second, and stir together the bread crumbs and smoked paprika in the third. Coat the chicken pieces in the flour, then dip fully in the egg. Dredge in the paprika bread crumbs, then transfer to a wire rack set over a baking sheet and spray both sides liberally with cooking spray.

2. Transfer 2 of the chicken cutlets to the air fryer oven. Select the Air Fry function and cook at 350 degrees Fahrenheit (177 degrees Celsius) for 6 minutes, or until beginning to brown. Spread each cutlet with 2 tablespoons of the marinara sauce and sprinkle with one-quarter of the smoked Mozzarella.
3. Increase the temperature to 400 degrees Fahrenheit (204 degrees Celsius) and air fry for 5 minutes more, or until the chicken is cooked through and crisp and the cheese is melted and golden brown.
4. Transfer the cutlets to a plate, stack on top of each other, and place inside a bun.

Repeat with the remaining chicken cutlets, marinara, smoked Mozzarella, and bun.

5. Serve the sandwiches warm.

Nutrition: Calories 311 Fat 11g Carbohydrate 22g Protein 31g

www.ingramcontent.com/pod-product-compliance
Lightning Source LLC
Chambersburg PA
CBHW070724030426
42336CB00013B/1910